NEIL FOSTER

Unleash Your Innner Fitness Warrior

Go from Bed to Gym & Smash your goals like a True Champion

First edition

This book was professionally typeset on Reedsy.
Find out more at reedsy.com

Contents

1   Introduction   1

2   The Fitness Warrior Mindset   6

3   Loving Yourself   14

4   Setting Goals   21

5   Conclusion   23

6   Resources   25

1

Introduction

Welcome Fitness Warriors my name is Neil Foster and I'm writing this book to deliver a very important message to you readers and listeners. I've been on my fitness journey for over a decade and I have given up, started again, failed, succeeded, felt unmotivated, and felt pointless. Because of my track record, I have come up with many different ways to still look and feel great which is the most important aspect despite my many failures. It doesn't have to be as tough as others make it. It's all in your mind. Think about your words. Your words were once thoughts that existed only in your mind. But when you open your mouth to speak, they become physical. If someone else hears those words, they start to develop into a perception of who you are. Words, actions and anything you express essentially is who you present yourself to be to the rest of the world. Fitness, like words, is a type of self expression. When you curl that 20 pound dumbbell, you are showing your mind that you can lift a 20 pound dumbbell. Your actions become a mirror and you start to feel like you are your actions. You are your words. You are a fitness warrior.

It's difficult to feel that way if you haven't stepped foot in a gym. However, I bet you can find yourself in other disciplines that resonate with your soul. For instance, if you think you're a lazy unmotivated person, you'll see others being that way and feel more content in your ways. If you feel that you are a smart person, you'll feel validated when you are around smart people. Like attracts to like. This doesn't always have to be a physical thing either. You can easily just entertain the thought of being a gym rat, an intellectual, or an overweight individual. When you see these things you start to feel either that it's an impossible feat, or that you can do that too.

Why You should Care about Fitness

I remember growing up with my brother and we'd be so interested in video games. We would level up our characters to embark on new missions, to receive even greater rewards and progress in the game. Fitness is somewhat the same. Think of your favorite video game. Runescape, Grand Theft Auto, Wizard 101 etc. In these types of games, you play as an avatar and can practically do whatever you want within the bounds of the game. You can make money by buying cars, property, and you can create businesses, alliances etc. However, pay attention to the part where you can take what's in your mind and essentially become what you visualize in the game through a series of challenges and hard work. Personally, I'm not much of a gamer, so my character isn't as highly skilled as some. However, for the little achievements I do have, I worked and played missions to accomplish the goals and buy the cars, and property I desired to gain an edge over other characters in the game.

Fitness isn't about gaining edges over other people. In my opinion you should leave your ego at the door. However, all of the same concepts can be applied to real life. You are your own avatar. Your mind, your body, and your spirit. Our thoughts, our words, are all manifested from your brain. You think, you speak. You think, you become. Fitness allows you to feel better physically and mentally. You will experience less muscle aches due to your strengths. The soreness that comes with pushing your body, becomes the reward, because you know that you're leveling up. Fitness allows you to be perceived differently to the world. Now that hot summer body attracts opportunities that you wouldn't otherwise have had. It brings an immeasurable amount of confidence, which allows you to get out of the house and to that beach, to that grocery store, to that music festival where you meet all types of people from all walks of life.

I'm not saying that you can't achieve this without fitness, but it's a catalyst. Fitness has been known to lower anxiety and cortisol levels, which reduces stress. On top of feeling better mentally, you will look and feel better. Walking up those stairs will start to feel easy. Running a mile wont feel like all hells breaking loose. You don't have to look like Arnold Schwarzenegger to feel like fitness has worked for you. Even just a simple 15-20 min short circuit workout has been known to improve your mental and physical capabilities.

Why You should care about Your Body

YOLO is what the kids say these days before they plunge themselves into a risky decision that could have dire consequences. You only get one life to live. Many individuals find themselves complaining about their lives and struggling to accept what they have been offered. Some have sacrificed themselves for others, and that is truly a blessing. However, I want you to understand that you have the right to be whoever you want. If you can dream it you can do it. It goes back to those words again. If you can think of it you can say it. If you can believe it, you can be it.

I understand that these phrases may sound corny and washed out. But I want you to understand that all these goals boil down to the choices and things that you tell yourself. If you can complain about being overweight, making jokes about how fat you are, and thinking it's pretty, then you can do the total opposite and speak life into your situation. Water yourself and water those around you. Spread positivity.

If you can put yourself in YOLO situations, give your life to your 9-5, sacrifice for your significant other, then why do you have to suffer in your own misery. Life tells us we must look out for our neighbor and not be too big on ourselves. But then you are the one that doesn't rise to your own dreams.

I'm not here to tell you to care about your body, because if you bought this book it's clear that you already do. I just want you to understand that you have to speak life to yourself, if you desire change. You have to make a choice and decide that this isn't you anymore. You get tired of being tired and one day you decide to make that change.

It may not be today that you make that change, but I would like to at least plant a seed within your mind that grows and enables you chase whatever fitness goals or desires you may have. It's all a feedback loop. Your mind follows your body and your body follows your mind.

What this book has to offer

In this book, I don't expect perfection from you. I don't want you to feel like a loser either. I just want to show you a different perspective on goal chasing. When you wake up and you pick up that iPhone to scroll through social media, you don't even think about it. If you stopped scrolling would you feel like a loser? you've never thought about that have you? That's because it's attached to you. It became who you are. That's what I want you to feel with fitness. I want it to become a part of your identity. You don't force it, you don't punish yourself. You simply be and allow what's in you to come to fruition in the physical world.

That is not an easy task, but life isn't easy either. You have no issue going to work, paying useless tickets and bills, just to be able to breathe at the end of the day. And everything you want and desire is on hold because of what? Other people's opinions, what the news says you must be. What social media says you must be.

Inside each and every one of us is greatness and that's what I want you to understand. You are already a fitness warrior because you're fighting a cause that matters to you whether you know it or not. If you bought this book, fitness obviously matters in some sense of the word. So in my eyes you are already a conqueror. Now it's your turn to believe it.

After completing this book I would like all of my readers and listeners to feel that whatever goals that they have in fitness, (whether that be to lose weight, gain weight, put on muscle, recomp, etc), that it is already in you to do these things. You just have to believe it to achieve it.

2

The Fitness Warrior Mindset

Why you are a Fitness Warrior

For a while, after I was terminated from my corporate tech job amidst my terrible breakup, I was so depressed that I couldn't get out of my bed. My dishes in the sink would stay there for weeks. I had to throw plates out because it got moldy from me not washing dishes and cleaning the food off. And you could say "Neil, how could you let all of that happen?" Something as simple as taking care of daily tasks, became difficult when my mind gave out due to life circumstances. I became a victim and I was depressed.

Funny enough before then, I was the total opposite. I was successful, living on my own in NYC at 23. I had my own apartment, had a decent girlfriend, went out with my friends and had a blast. Throughout all of that I was a serious gym rat. I couldn't miss a workout, I ate so much bulked up and looked totally different from my skinny self. My friends were complimenting me and it felt great. But it all came crashing down when life decided to take it away from me.

For those months that felt like years, I never thought I'd completely abandon everything that I'd once identified with. The gym, the girls, the fast life I was living it all became pointless. I became a social recluse and I barely ate anything. I still question to this day, how I didn't really lose much of my gains considering my diet, and my lack of activity.

But during this time, I was still a warrior. The fight became different. It was spiritual, mental and physical warfare, everyday. Yes, me laying down in my bed became a fight of the mind as much as going to my physically demanding job, became a fight of the body.

I bet you could relate to some of this. You fight in ways that you may not even know. For example, you may have to deal with irrational people in the workplace, maybe something as simple as getting out of the bed every morning to head to work, taking your kids to school, showing up in life with a smile, paying bills. It's all a fight and we have been conditioned to think this is normal. Technically, it is, because that's the modern world. However, those dreams you have and hold onto still exist and they must come to fruition. That same fight it takes to not cause a fit during serious traffic jams, is the same emotional intelligence and control, you can apply to get in the gym.

You may say Neil, if I'm working hard and taking care of the kids and sacrificing my life for others, how can I even make time or even remotely have the energy to exercise? Well, you have to understand that everything in life is a choice. You can do whatever you please, but regret is a strong indicator that you're not living in alignment with your goals. You should never feel bad that it took longer than expected to get on your grind however. It's all about staying in momentum and building your strength to ultimately crush anything you desire.

It's about putting yourself first even if for 23 hrs you think about others and what you're conditioned to believe you need to survive. You can literally walk to the gym and walk out in 2 minutes. Yes, that may not feel like much, but you made it to the gym, and you put your goals first. Not your bills, not your fears, but yourself. Your dreams, your vision. That's who.

The Fitness Warrior Mentality

The fitness warrior mentality is something we all innately have. As a toddler you learned to walk right? Well that same determination it took to try again until you got it right is the same willpower you will use to develop your fitness mindset. Fitness is for everyone, and if you want to crush your goals, you have to understand that it's already in you to achieve them. It's all about aligning yourself to that vibration of energy. Maybe you feel that you don't need to workout. You can get through the day just fine. I've had those thoughts when it came to me working out and going to the boxing gym at the same time. I felt the gym was useless. However, if you can drink yourself to death, or smoke a joint till you smoke out, or watch Netflix until you feel like you're the main character in the script, then you can develop yourself.

You never know why you have that urge. That urge to succeed, the urge to get that body. Maybe if you get that body, maybe you'll say to yourself, "I don't deserve to live paycheck to paycheck. If I can get the body of my dreams, I can get the money of my dreams." Maybe one day, you're walking around with your muscular chest at the beach, and someone comes up to you and offers you a modeling opportunity. Your 9-5 job, that you've grown to despise, disappears in the neverland. A more realistic and more valuable outcome however, is how the mindset starts to apply to your life. You stop settling for being the fat guy, you stop settling for those types of girls or guys because you feel like you're entitled to more. And I know that sounds bad, because no one is better than anyone, but you will find more alignment within your life if you decide to put yourself first and find out what you are really capable of.

Past failures and the Victim Mentality

In life, we are guaranteed to go through ups and downs. Look at the planet we live on. Earth has gone through various changes to be what it is today. We see what is presented and it may not be perfect, but it's normal to us. Once upon a time during the Triassic Period, the continents were once one large piece of land known as Pangea. This island was surrounded by water. In modern times, that same section of land has separated and created what we know as continents. Throughout these changes, which ended a few animal species the Earth was reborn. This modification reintroduced different cultures, experiences and lifetimes. Now everyone has a different story, upbringing, dialect, etc. This only adds to our experience in life. It may not be perfect but it sure is interesting don't you think?

We have all gone through failures. If you haven't, then I don't think you have lived enough, because it does happen. Even when applying for jobs you will experience rejection. However, all that salt and dirt life has been thrown at you, can at least be used to build a fort. Something you can call your own. Even if it's made out of dirt, it's still yours and you own it. We own our experiences that's what makes us who we are. These ups and downs enable us to feel great when we reach our goals. A sunny day wouldn't feel as great if it happened everyday. And as 50 cent says in his song "Many Men", "Joy wouldn't feel so good if it wasn't for pain". It's true, and when we reach that joy, we can give back to others that are stuck in their pain. This will enable us as a human collective to move forward as we reach out and help others.

Some people never leave the victim mindset. It's not easy. Life can be extremely brutal to some. However, you own it and must take responsibility for it. We have no issue accepting the highs of life, even if it's purely chance or luck. You would want to think that you influenced the outcome, and maybe you did. On the flipside, when it's cloudy and things aren't going your way that's purely life being life. Evolution as you may say. All the extra weight and mental burdens that you carry must disappear during this season if you expect to be refined into the beautiful gem you already are. If you get rejected from 1000 jobs, you've learned 1000 ways to take a no. You've learned 1000 ways to complain as well, and you realize that those 1000 complaints aren't going to give you a paycheck. So you must cease the complaints and focus on 1000 different ways to make it.

Do you give up? Some might. But you don't, because you have the Fitness Warrior mindset, You push through because you have bills to pay. You have to put food in your mouth, and you have to maintain a place to live. So if we can condition ourselves to care about societal needs then, why can't you do the same when it comes to your goals?

Setting Your Eyes on the Vision

A lot of times, you need a vision. It isn't something that is easy to have when all there is chaos around. Maybe you want to be able to walk up the stairs without breathing so hard. Maybe you want to be able to lift your groceries with ease as you bring them to your car, without assistance. It could be as simple as that. It starts with a little vision. Take a few minutes to think about what you want. Imagine it as deeply as you can. See it as if it's already who you are. If you can't imagine it, then surround yourself with it. Find pictures of the body you want. Search videos on Youtube that demonstrate the types of activities you would like to do with your body. After you get that image, really try to focus on it in your mind space. See yourself with that 6 pack, walking on the beach and the girls are looking. See yourself wearing that beautiful dress you saw window shopping at the clothing store. If you have the funds, buy the dress, touch the dress, feel the dress. Really become acquainted with you and what you want to be. Once that baseline is set, you've already accomplished it. It goes back to thoughts and manifesting words. If you can think it, you can say it, and if you can say it, it becomes a part of your perception of who you are.

I want you to understand that what you're doing when you are visualizing, is that you are changing your perception of things that you desire and making it yours. Instead of the object being something to chase, it's who you already are. Instead of you thinking that you're a fat slob, you imagine that you are a beach body model. Because you've imagined it, it becomes who you are. It becomes a part of you.

Block Out Distractions

The last section sounds easy, when you read it. But you'll quickly see that just because you've imagined it doesn't mean you're there. The goal shouldn't be to reach your goal. Your goal is to change how you view the goal. It's to make it attainable. That's who you are.

However, we have to make some physical changes to things around us. We have to cut things out that we don't need. For instance, would a lady wearing that dress, be eating ice cream everyday, and skipping their workouts? Hmm maybe, and maybe that's the way you can go. You could even try it for a week and see how that works for you. Let reality determine that for you. I really want you to see for yourself how things work for your body and mind. Because, there are people out there that can get away with certain things others can't. It's not a simple 1 2 3 step by step rule book. I'm trying to get you to understand that everyone is different and that you should really try things out instead of adhering to a script that doesn't resonate with your soul.

Once you see that this can't work, and you don't like the way something feels, you can begin to trim things that don't align with what YOU FEEL is not going to get you any closer to that goal. I've literally read all types of books, and articles to help me in my life, and what I've realized is

I'm the type that has to learn by my own experience. Some things may work in the short term, but it really comes down to the question "Does this fit with who I am fundamentally?" This may seem to contradict what I was saying earlier but if you think about it, not everyone wants to do things the same way. We're all bred differently, and if it doesn't align with your spirit it will not align with your goals or vision. You will be forcing yourself into something that requires more energy than just doing said thing because that's who I am. You can try if that something sticks, then great. For instance if you realize I need my ice cream, then limit your intake of it but still do what needs to be done. Maybe, you have to work harder just to achieve your goals just because you won't sacrifice the ice cream. That's all up to how you want to live.

Incremental Exposure

After you've decided that you needed to cut some things out, try to add some things in. For instance, for me to fit in this dress, I need to hit the gym at least 3 times a week. Now from being a slouch in the bed like I was watching the 700th tarot video on YouTube about drama, to going outside, seeing people and going to the gym it may seem like a stretch. So make it easier for yourself. Instead of taking the train or driving your car, maybe you sacrifice $10 for a cab ride so you can prepare yourself mentally for a workout. Maybe, instead of going to the gym you decide to just say I'm going to do one push up a day. Yes! I said it just one. It may not seem like much but you have to start where you are. You could literally eat a scoop of ice cream, sit down and watch your favorite show and say I'm going to do one push up when there is a commercial. This is an example of how much you should break your goals down.

Now instead of you eating the ice cream, you can now add that you do one push up. Already, you can see how that changes the paradigm. You could do that for as long as you desire. However, we have goals to reach, and eventually you will feel the need to add on more. Maybe you do two push ups. Maybe you put a crunch in there every now and then. The point is, you are telling your mind by doing this that I want more. It's only natural for your mind to seek greater and your options on achieving your goals will expand. It all starts with just a little bit of faith in yourself and the world.

3

Loving Yourself

Understanding that you deserve your dream body

In my opinion, two types of people exist. There is the person who thinks they can and those who can't. It is one thing to be humble and know your place and role in society. However, if you constantly find yourself sacrificing and putting your dreams last and needs and wants others first, do you truly and deeply love yourself? Think about your child if you have one, or anything you value deeply. You would want that person, place or thing to grow and maintain itself. Would you want your child to grow up and not know basic self care, how to maintain a job. You would instill future lessons to that child. That's what you have to do for yourself. It isn't about that bill that you need to pay. There will always be bills. It isn't about taking a bite out of that cake because there will always be cake. It's about loving yourself enough that you think about the future, aka the successful version of you, as you would your child. All of that love builds up, and it essentially becomes that child's inner version of themselves.

As life progresses, traumatic things do happen, and it may cause you to take breaks on important life aspects. You may feel you need these things the most. However during these breaks, you learn what matters most. It's to not lose yourself in the madness. When you get back in the world, you double down on what makes you you even if it wasn't you before.

You are entitled to do whatever you want in this world. There will be naysayers, jealous people, haters, but you have to understand that you matter to you. If you feel called to have the body of your dreams then you go get it despite what anybody says. You owe you.

You are the One

These days, everyone gets inspired and wants to copy celebrities and social media influencers and become the identical to each other because they want the same attention. There's nothing wrong with that at all, that's the way of life now. However, you need to understand that you are the best guide you have. If you bought this book, you have it in you to create your own superhero, which is who you are in your mind. That's who you try to become. I remember scrolling through social media in my college days and I saw a video of a roller skater listening to Peter Rock skating down the city streets. I thought it looked amazing. I wanted it to be me.I wanted to experience that. It wasn't until a couple of years later that I saw that video again. This time, my mindset was different, I had been through enough that I felt that I could be and do whatever I wanted. I literally saw myself in that video. I saw myself with those roller skates on, even though as a kid I completely gave up on the idea. I tried it maybe once or twice as a 8 year old boy, then quickly grew out of them and thought I could never go back. This time however was different. I thought I could never lose my financial stability even though I worked so hard to achieve it. I never thought I could be the butt of jokes in my friend groups because of lies spread on my name. I never thought after applying so much effort to attract women, that I would not want them as much once I saw the effects of being in a toxic relationship. So if all of these things happened to me and I didn't ask for it, why couldn't I get the things that I asked for?

So one day, I just bought my inline skates and headed to the skate park, in the crack of winter at 20 odd degree weather and said "I'm going to be able skate by the summer". Sure enough, I became good at it, and was having a blast. However, it all started with me and a decision to just do it. That's exactly how you will begin what seems impossible. It's seeing and then believing.

If it's in your reality it's for you

Something that I don't see stressed enough in the world is how your surroundings really do influence you. Yes, if you hang with the wrong crowd you'll become what they are. The top 5 people you hang around will influence you. I get all that. I understand. However, there are things outside of what you directly interact with that can influence you as well. We just take it however we feel at that moment. We may not give it a second thought. For instance, when I was running low in my bank account, all I'd see were expensive cars. I was drawn to them and they were drawn to me. I didn't hate, I didn't feel jealous but I knew that I couldn't have it at that moment delivering food in 20 degree weather, high winds and snow. I just stayed on my course and kept making my under minimum wage check, with barely any tips. However, that next month I got a callback from a job that would literally give me back everything that I lost. With that job, I was able to get a car. Now, it's not a Lamborghini, or Maserati, but it does attract attention. I'm not much of an attention seeker, to the point that I wanted to sell it, to keep a lower profile, but I kept it.

This situation showed me that I can see things in my reality and they are there for a reason. So for an overweight person who wants to lose weight. Maybe one day, you are buying groceries and at the self checkout, you see someone buying healthier food options. You are seeing that for a reason. Don't think it's a coincidence. It's in your reality, so it's going to be you if you want it to be. Now, some take that energy, begin to hate and think, "Who does this guy think he is?". The judgemental person feels like they should be eating healthier subconsciously but they don't want to or can't so they despise anyone who can. The world makes it easier for people like this to feel justified in their beliefs because these days, everybody is a winner. That's great, but do you believe that you are a winner, that's what matters. If you feel repulsed by someone else and their choices, how they look or how they act, maybe it's a reflection upon you, your choices and what you don't like about yourself. Like I said if you picked this book, you already desire a change. So, whether or not you want to put in the work is up to you, but notice what you feel triggered or inspired by.

Maybe you feel inspired by seeing a beach model, and you feel that that's not who you want to be and that's okay but if it makes you feel a certain way, then you have to ask why. Then proceed to make those changes, because the world is only here to make you into whatever it wants you to be or who you want to be. Don't be fooled by the illusions.

Treat Yourself

All work, no play, isn't for the weak. When I'd work at my job, I don't remember a "thank you", or a "congratulations" from anybody. But I sure do remember joining a meeting one day, to be told randomly that I was terminated. Because of this, I was unable to get an unemployment check. The city denied me. So from that point on, I decided to celebrate myself. No one really cares about what you do. It doesn't matter how much work or effort you put in, you can't guarantee that it will be received by others. Because of this, you have to treat yourself.

I remember when I was putting together my first Airbnb Arbitrage unit, and I was met with so many unique challenges. I never pictured any of the things that happened. None of what I was taught was my experience. It was tougher to put together and I took longer than any of the other participants in the community that I was in. Nonetheless, I got it done. Afterwards, I took myself to *Outback Steakhouse* and ordered the biggest steak on the menu. It was so interesting because the waitress kept calling me boss. I didn't think much of it, but I definitely needed to hear that, because I felt like I was constantly having the rug pulled from under me, losing and failing, spending unnecessary money and being taken advantage of. Nevertheless, a boss is what I was becoming. So even from treating myself to something as simple as a steak, the world rewarded me even more just for rewarding myself. I felt honored by the world even though I was eating food by myself. You may read this and think that it sounds arrogant to assume, but it's not about what the person said, it's about how you receive it. If someone uttered something bad about you, you wear it, so why not wear the compliments.

Failure

During your journey to become more active, you will experience a fatigue in motivation. You won't want to leave bed, you won't care about doing that push-up after your ice cream. You may feel like it is pointless. Maybe, it is. Maybe it is pointless, but you have to remember why you started. You have to remember that the quicker you get something the quicker you lose it. Rewards aren't the reason that you should embark on a journey in the first place, it should be something that you do because you want to. You started this because you saw that 6 pack in your vision. You started this because you wanted to be confident in your own skin. You didn't like feeling your thighs rubbing together when you walked. You didn;'t like feeling tired after walking a block to the store to get a nicotine pod, or a pack of cigarettes. So you made a decision to be the best that you can be so why stop now?

I'm not here to tell you that failure doesn't happen. You'll skip workouts, you'll entertain things you shouldn't, however that's what makes you the strong fitness warrior that you are. It's about how you handle the rain and when you don't feel like it. Okay, you skip a day, are you going to go back the next day? It's not about earning back what you lost, it's about recreating the present. Instead of worrying and feeling regretful, simply tell yourself, it won't happen again. If it does, tell yourself again. It's not easy to be a machine, because we're not. Life happens, and you feel like everything may be pointless to try, because of bumps in the road. But that's the whole point. That's what builds the character. That's what makes you humble, and that my friend is what keeps you going.

Being Humble

Fast results breed an ego. As much as I would like to tell you that, you can flip on a switch and be successful, or that everything you want is a linear progression would be crazy. Life is an up and down game. It isn't fair and can be ruthless to some. All we own are our experiences. You don't own the results. You don't own that 6 pack just because it's on your body. You don't own your stamina, your fatigue, your results. Because as quick or as slow as you got them, it could be taken all away. Accidents happen, and it's unfortunate. That's why it's always good to be humble and be grateful for even having all that you have. Being humble also goes into not shaming yourself for missing a workout. Okay big deal, you missed a workout. Don't place so much importance on it. Be grateful that you missed it, maybe that is the day you would have pulled a tendon, or had an accident in the gym. Things happen, and things happen for a reason. If the world is trying to teach a lesson, it will make sure that you learn one way or another. So always be grateful. Okay, you are overweight, but you still have your limbs. Okay, you skipped a workout, but you still have food to eat, and can cook and prepare the food. Don't be so hard on yourself, because it can all be taken away in a flash.

4

Setting Goals

Make a list of what you want to achieve in fitness

Goal setting is very important. You may divert from your goals for years, but as long as you have them, you can stay sane and know that you are working towards something. Look around, and try to find yourself. What do you want out of this fitness journey? Do you want to be muscular, bulked, skinny, plus sized with a little tone. Whatever you decide, make a list. Doesn't have to be special at all. You don't need to buy a special journal or any hyped up tool. Just write it down somewhere.

When you write it down, think about how you can break it into chunks, manageable enough for you. Even if it's to get up and walk around your house for 1 minute a day. Just write it down and stick to it. If you forget, or don't feel like hitting that goal, then don't worry about it. It isn't something that should determine your self worth or make you feel like a loser because you failed. You should get up and try again, until it sticks. Truth be told, it may never stick but getting results is all about showing up. I'd skip workouts all the time when I was heavy into lifting weights. It never affected my overall results because the amount of work that I put in when I was present overshadowed all of the times I didn't show up. Just put your best foot forward everyday and show yourself that you can do it. It eventually stacks up and before you know it, you're curling 30 pounds at the gym. That may not seem impressive to you active gym goers, but retrofit what I said to your experience. For some, it's walking up a flight of stairs, or just walking. For others it's just to get just enough motivation to get to that next step. Maybe you have a 4 pack and want a 6 pack. Apply the knowledge as you see fit.

5

Conclusion

How you will move forward after this book

This book should have provided you with the proper mindset when attacking your fitness goals. It all starts within your mind. It's all a decision that you make for your well being. It isn't easy to stay on target all the time, but I hope that you recognize that if you can form thoughts and push your words into reality, then you can become fit. It's just about aligning your mind with your body, and pushing yourself when things are hard. It isn't easy but with enough failure which is always going to be expected, you will see the results eventually. Failure is there to keep you in check and accountable. Failure is enough, don't insult yourself. Love yourself, love your body for making a decision for you. At the end of the day, we don't own any of the results, only the character building and the experiences we have while on the journey to greatness.

How to implement what you learned

You might have found a few points in this book that have resonated with you. Take those thoughts, own them and implement them. This book was to provide an alternative way of crushing goals. Instead of thinking of goals as an upward climb, look at it more as fusing your life with other activities to become what you were already destined to be. If you see it, it's already you. If you can believe it you can achieve it. It all starts in the mind and your body is just a tool to achieve and align with your mind. So with that said Fitness Warriors set out on their own missions to achieve greatness in this world. You owe to yourself and yourself only. Start somewhere, anywhere. Remember your attitude is your altitude so keep it positive.

Much love Neil Foster.

If you found the book helpful please leave a favorable review on Amazon, it is much appreciated :)

Best Wishes on Your Fitness Journey!

6

Resources

Bailey, B. (2016, June 18). *Leave everything in God's hands - wisdom Hunters.* Wisdom Hunters. https://www.wisdomhunters.com/leave-everything-gods-hands/

Blain, T., MA. (2024, April 30). *Why is it important to stay humble?* Verywell Mind. https://www.verywellmind.com/why-is-it-important-to-be-humble-5223266#:~:text=Being%20humble%20allows%20one%20to,and%20who%20they%20are%20not.

Depression and anxiety: Exercise eases symptoms. (2023, December 23). Mayo Clinic. https://www.mayoclinic.org/diseases-conditions/depression/in-depth/depression-and-exercise/art-20046495#:~:text=Regular%20exercise%20may%20improve%20depression,them%20over%20the%20long%20term.

GotQuestions.org. (2022, January 4). *GotQuestions.org.* https://www.gotquestions.org/power-of-words.html

Harvard Health. (2020, July 7). *Exercising to relax.* https://www.health.harvard.edu/staying-healthy/exercising-to-relax#:~:text=The%20me

ntal%20benefits%20of%20aerobic,natural%20painkillers%20and%20 mood%20elevators.

Lisaparziale. (2023, February 6). *The power of visualization: imagining yourself doing something helps you achieve your goal - Rowan Center for Behavioral Medicine.* Rowan Center for Behavioral Medicine. https://ww w.rowancenterla.com/the-power-of-visualization-imagining-yourself -doing-something-helps-you-achieve-your-goal/

Sharratt, L. (2021, November 14). *How to Make Peace with the Past and Stop Being a Victim.* Tiny Buddha. https://tinybuddha.com/blog/how-to- make-peace-with-the-past-and-stop-being-a-victim/

The Earth through time. (n.d.). https://www.gsi.ie/en-ie/education/our- planet-earth/Pages/The-Earth-through-time.aspx

What was Pangea? | U.S. Geological Survey. (2009, February 10). https://www.usgs.gov/faqs/what-was-pangea#:~:text=At%20the% 20beginning%20of%20the,this%20supercontinent%20slowly%20bro ke%20apart.